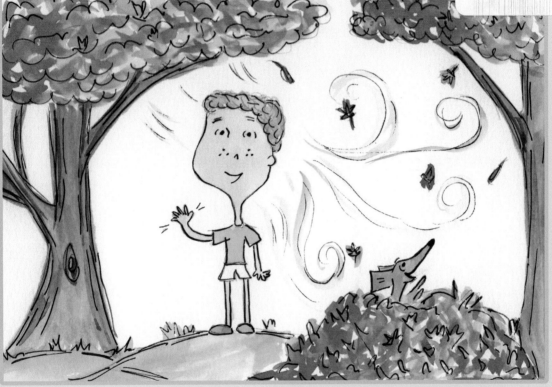

Hi there! I have cystic fibrosis–'CF' for short. I was born
with it just like I was born with blond hair, green eyes,
and a million tiny freckles. CF comes from a gene
that your parents pass down to you.

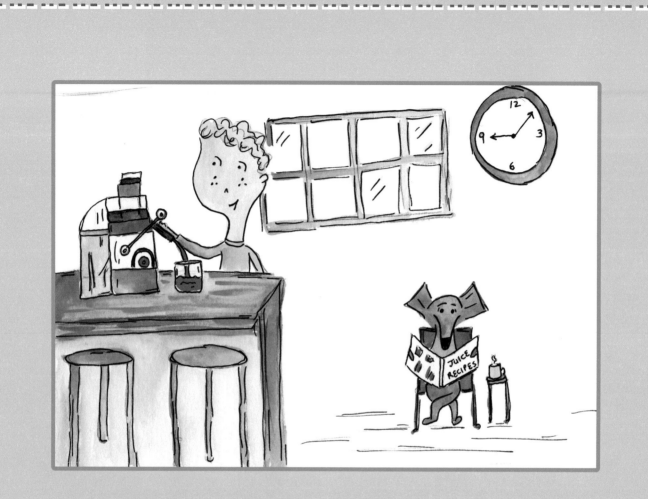

So, what is CF and what does it do? Great questions!
It took me a while to understand it so it's okay to get confused.
I like to think of it as a problem with our juice machines.

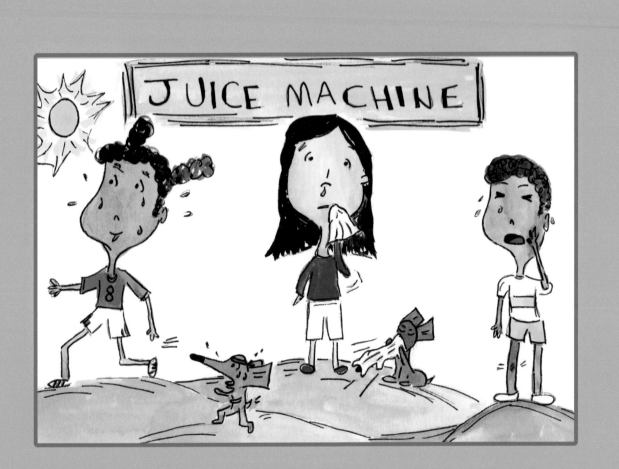

Our bodies are juice machines. Sounds silly, I know.
But our bodies make juices every second of every minute of
every day! Our juice machine churns out sweat (yuck), mucus
(more yuck), and tears (for sad days). We even make special
digestive juices to break down foods we eat.

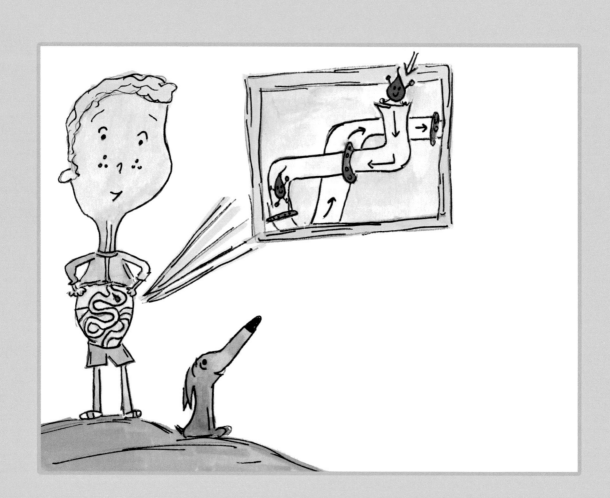

Our juices must travel through our body's system of pipes to do their jobs. So, they have to be thin, slick, and fast – just like juice you sip through a straw. Slurrrrpppppp.

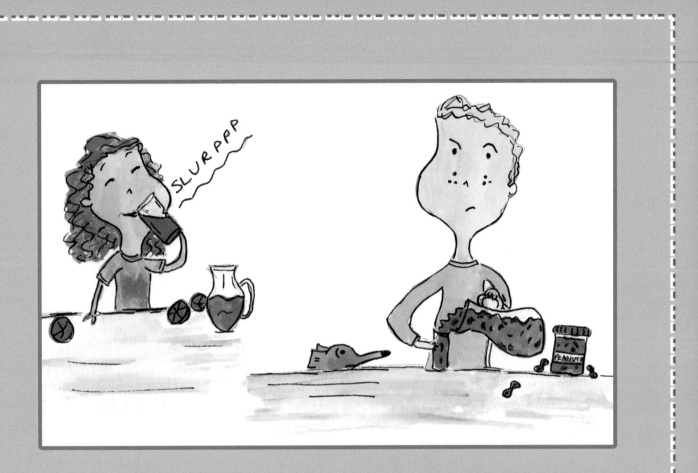

Now in CF, our juice machines act a little different. We still make the same types of juices, but instead of being thin and slick, our juices can be thick and sticky. Instead of being like flowing orange juice, our juices may be thick like sticky caramel. Instead of being like smooth pineapple juice, our juices may be as chunky as a peanut butter sundae.

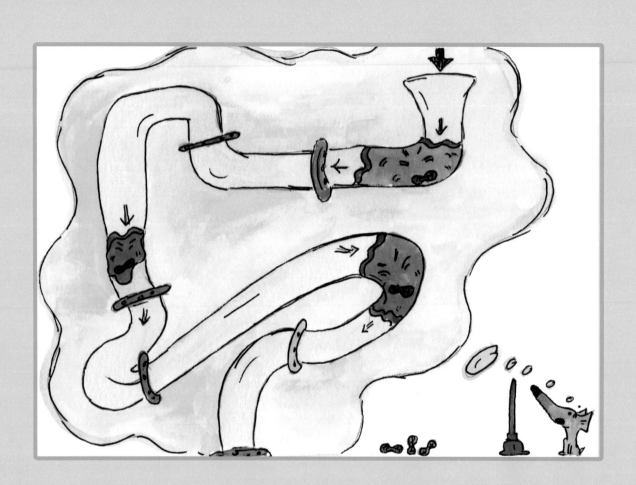

Our juices are so thick and clumpy that they can get stuck in our body's system of pipes. And then they can't do their jobs. Imagine trying to slurp up caramel through a straw. Not easy!

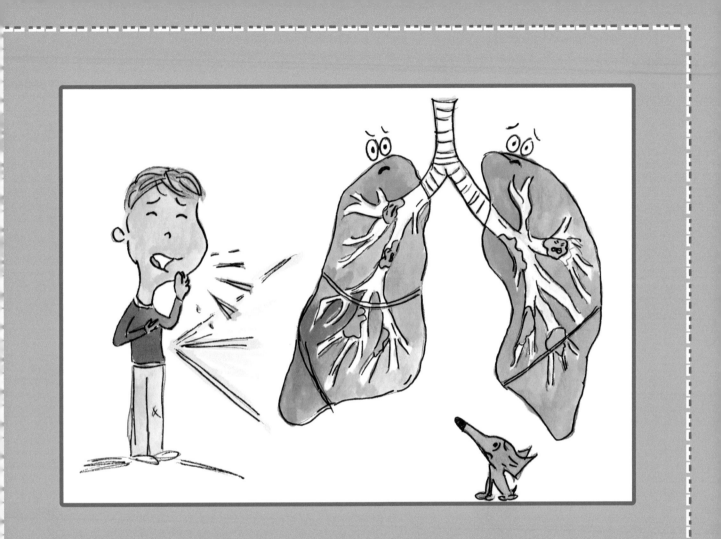

Mucus, the juice in our lungs, can become so thick that it can get stuck anywhere from our nose to deep in our lungs. It can make it hard for us to breathe. It can make us cough, cough, and cough some more. It can hurt our lungs and it can make us sick.

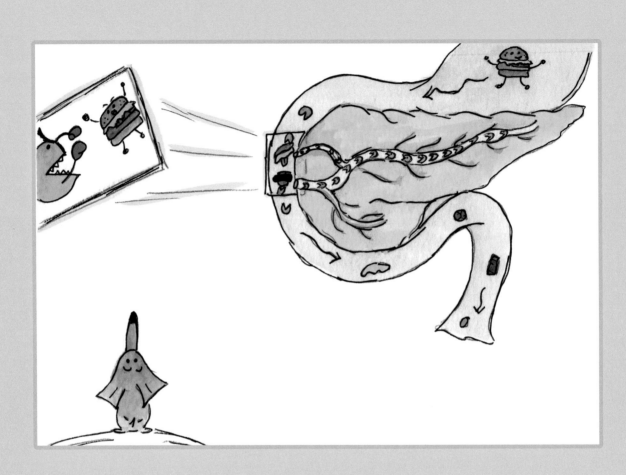

Our pancreas can get in trouble too. Our pancreas is a funny-looking, corn-shaped organ that makes digestive juices. These juices contain enzymes, which are special proteins that break down the food we eat—like juicy burgers! This helps us digest our food and grow big and strong!

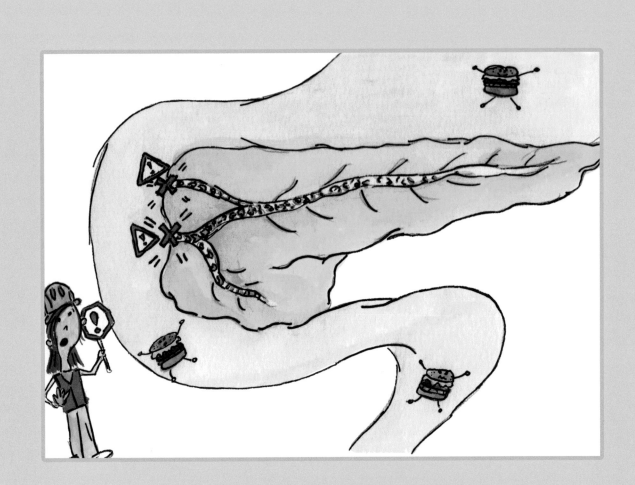

Sometimes with CF, our enzymes can get stuck in our pancreas. This means no matter how many juicy burgers we eat, we may not gain weight. This can also make us sick.

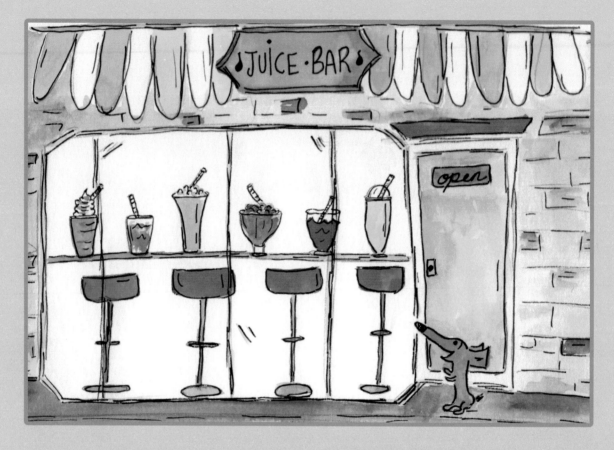

So, do all of our juice machines act the same in CF? Nope! All juice machines are different. So, while my juice machine may make thick pancreas juices, yours may make only thick mucus. But don't worry! No matter how your juice machine works, there are lots of treatments to help our thick, clumpy juices. Let's start with our lungs.

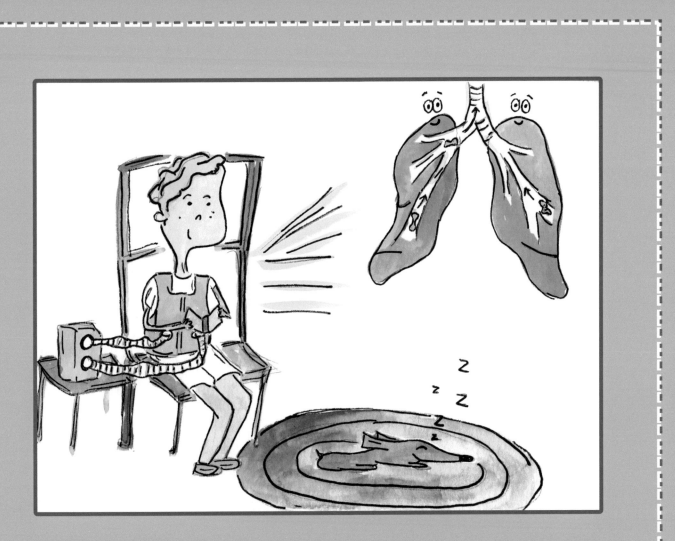

Special breathing treatments help us break up our chunky, sticky mucus so we can get it out of our lungs. Goodbye mucus! This is an important job. We have to remember to do it every day. And in the right order too!

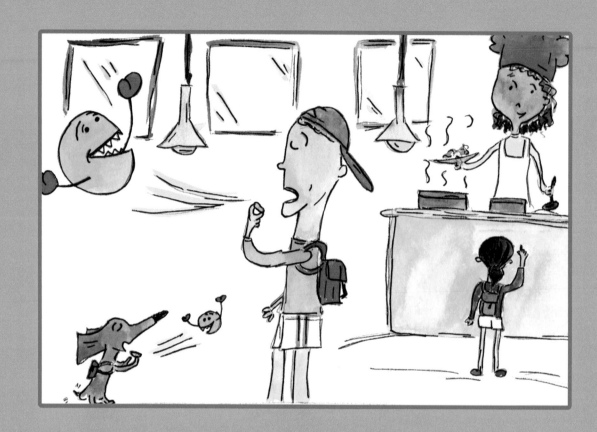

Next, call in the enzymes! Since our enzymes get stuck in our pancreas with our digestive juices, we need to take replacement ones. These replacement enzymes replace our stuck ones so we can still break down our food giving us the nutrition we need. Taking them before we eat every meal is important so we can grow big and strong!

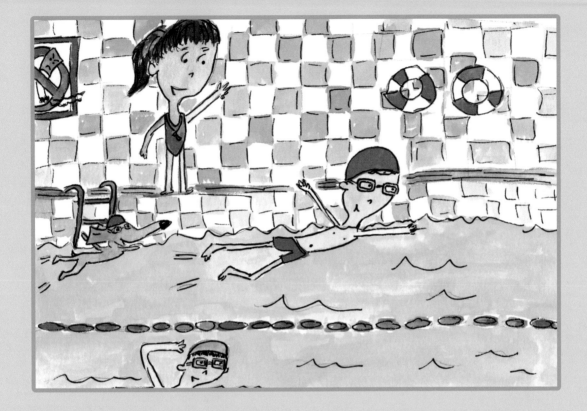

Exercise and diet are also important ways to fight our thick, clumpy juices. Special medicines from our doctors also work to protect us. As can staying far away from cigarette smoke (big yuck!)

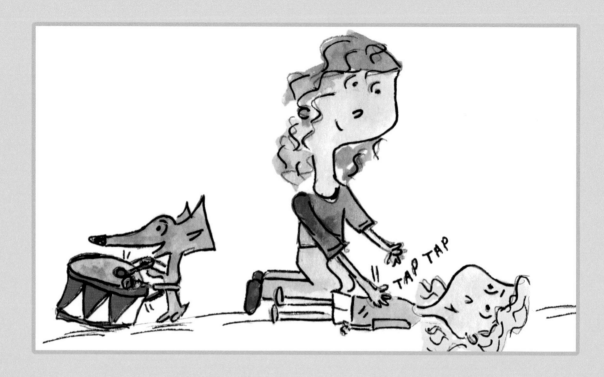

See, there are ways to help our wacky juice machines. It does take extra work and extra strength. But we are strong! And most importantly, we are not alone!

# Facts

CF is a lifelong disease that does not have a cure...YET!

CF is different in everyone! It can affect one body part, two body parts, or many. It acts differently in each one of us, which makes each of our stories and treatments unique!

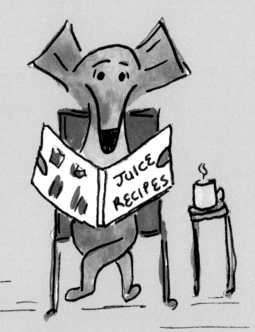

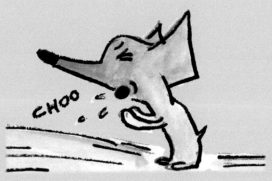

CF is not contagious! Just because we may cough a lot, this does not mean we can make anyone near us sick from CF.

You are not alone! There are tens of thousands of us living with CF. That's a lot of wacky juice machines...

CF is an **autosomal recessive** genetic disorder. It means both of your parents have to have a **mutation** in a gene in order for you to get CF.

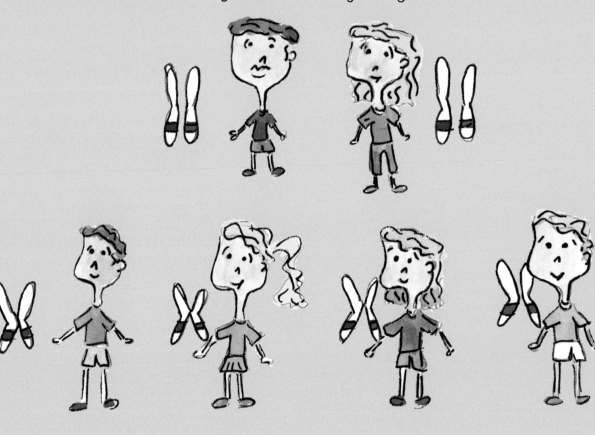

Although CF is most common in people of European ancestry, it occurs in all ethnic groups.

Every baby who is born in the United States gets a **screening test** for CF. If this test is positive, a **sweat test** is done to confirm the **diagnosis**.

Most children with CF are diagnosed with **newborn screening** in the first few months of their lives. CF can still be diagnosed in older kids who may not have had newborn screening. Thankfully, there are only a few mutations that a newborn screen may not identify.

CF causes our bodies to make a protein that is abnormal.

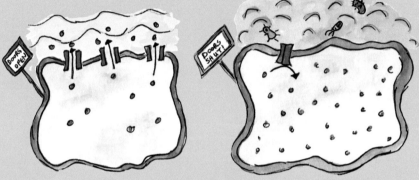

This irregular protein is what causes all of our juices to get very thick and sticky, instead of thin and watery. It makes doors shut in our cells, which leads to our mucus becoming thick.

Our thick, sticky juices trap bacteria in our lungs causing our lungs to get sick and often infected. They can block our pancreas so we cannot break down the vitamins and nutrients in our food. They can also affect our liver, sweat glands, and reproductive organs.

CF does not affect our brain. No juices get stuck up there!

# Common CF Symptoms

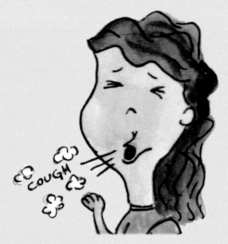

- Lots and lots of coughing with thick mucus
- Skin that tastes salty (like the ocean!)
- Getting sick often from respiratory infections (like colds, bronchitis, or pneumonia)

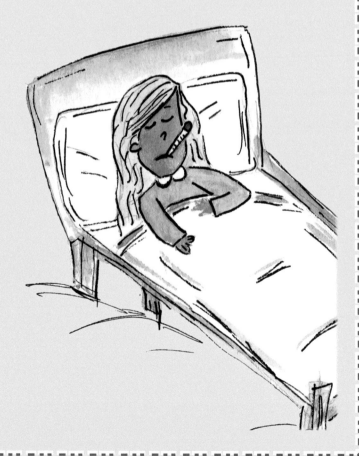

- Feeling short of breath and wheezing
- Having trouble growing even though you're eating
- Having lots of poops that look greasy

# Airway Clearance

This is how we can help keep our lungs healthy and clear. There are lots of different airway clearance therapies!

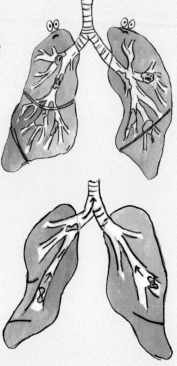

**Percussion and postural drainage (P&PD) –** this is also called **chest physical therapy**. It's when you let gravity and clapping help drain your mucus. You sit or lie in different positions and then tap (or clap) your chest to help stuck mucus get knocked free. Sort of like pretending your body is a drum! Then cough all that mucus out!

TAP TAP

**Positive expiratory pressure (PEP) -** You use a special breathing tube that is easy to take a deep breath in, but difficult to take a deep breath out. This helps get air into your lungs and behind your stuck mucus to knock it free! You finish with a **huff cough**.

HUFF!

**Active cycle of breathing techniques (ACBT) –** This is different types of breathing that do three big things:

#1 **breathing control**. This relaxes your airway. Breathe in through your nose and out through your mouth with your lips smooched up like you're about to plant a big kiss!

#2 **chest expansion**. This helps get air behind your stuck mucus. Take a deep breath over 3-seconds. Then breathe out slowly and not forcefully. You can use chest clapping with this!

#3 **huff coughing**. This helps force your mucus out of your lungs! Deep slow breath in, HOLD IT, and then slowly exhale. Keep doing this until all your mucus is gone!

**Autogenic drainage (AD) –** this is a fancy word for 'self-drainage'. You change your breathing speed to help move your stuck mucus.

**Oscillatory PEP devices (OPEP) –** These devices shake up your lungs to help free mucus that is stuck. You blow out of the device a bunch of times to create the vibrations and then finish with a huff cough!

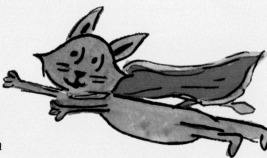

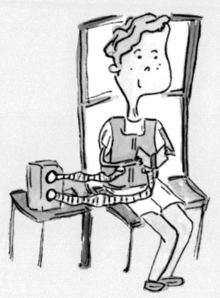

**High frequency chest compression (HFCC) –** You get to wear a fancy vest for this one! The vest shakes your chest and blows up like a balloon to help un-stick mucus from your lungs. After 5 minutes, don't forget to pause and huff cough that mucus out of there!

**Exercise. Exercise. Exercise.** This will always help your lungs!!

# Nutrition! Eat Up!

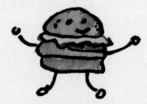

1. A good diet is super important in CF for lots of reasons:
   a. Helps us fight infections
   b. Helps our lungs grow, heal, and stay healthy
   c. Helps our bodies grow
2. We need **TWO TIMES** the calories that other kids our age need. This is because of malabsorption and our energy needs.
   a. **Malabsorption** is when our pancreatic enzymes are stuck and cannot break down our food. (see page 8-9!)
   b. Our energy needs are high because of all the breathing exercises we do to keep our lungs healthy.
3. So what should we eat?
   a. FATS, FATS, and more FATS!
   b. Lots of salt
   c. Lots of protein
   d. Pancreatic enzymes (see page 12)
   e. Vitamins

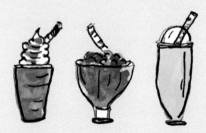

4. Sometimes even if we eat all the right food, we still need a little extra help to grow and gain weight. If we do, our doctor may give us nutritional supplements, or special drinks and snacks to help us get even more calories.

All about the enzymes:

1. 9 out of 10 of us need to take **pancreatic enzymes** (see page 12) that look like little pills.

2. Make sure to take them at the beginning of every meal and snack.

   a. The ONLY foods that you do NOT need to take enzymes for are:

i.   Fruits

ii.   Juice

iii.   Soft drinks

iv.   Sports drinks

v.   Tea & coffee (without cream!)

vi.   Hard candy

vii.   Fruit snacks

viii.   Jelly beans

ix.   Gum

x.   Popsicles

xi.   Flavored ice

3. Don't ever skip taking them! They help break down your food so you can use it for energy and to grow big and strong.

4. Keep your enzymes out of the hot sun and the freezing cold.

5. Most pancreatic enzymes come as a capsule with little beads. You can either swallow the capsule or, if you have trouble swallowing, you can open the capsule and mix the little beads into an acidic food like applesauce!

**And now bring in the modulators!**

Remember how in CF, our CF causes our bodies to make a protein (the **CFTR protein**) that is abnormal (see page 17)? Well, new medicines are being made that make that CFTR protein normal again. These are called **CFTR modulators**.

Some examples of these modulators are combinations of the following medicines: ivacaftor, lexacaftor, tezacaftor, and lumacaftor. Each one targets a specific type of gene mutation. So, it depends on which type of mutation you have, when deciding if you will need to take a modulator, and which one you will take!

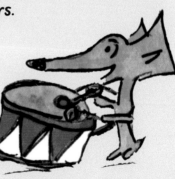

# Meet Your Team!

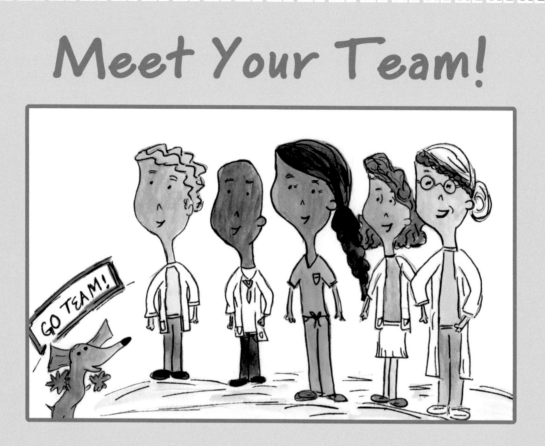

1. Your **lung doctor (pulmonologist)** is in charge of taking care of your lungs and keeping them healthy. You will see your lung doctor regularly.

2. Your **GI doctor (gastroenterologist)** is in charge of taking care of any problems with your intestines, liver, and stomach. You will see your GI doctor regularly.

3. Your **nurse navigator** or **program coordinator** is like your cruise ship director. They coordinate your entire care plan and make sure all your teams are communicating and on the same page. They will also teach you about CF and your care journey.

4. You may meet **nurse practitioners (NP)** and **physician's assistants (PA)** as well. They are partners with your CF doctors and are also in charge of taking care of you and teaching you about CF. You will see them regularly as well.

5. Your **social worker** helps you and your family with stress and emotions. They also help make sure you are able to get the care you need, when you need it.

6. Your **dietitian** helps you with your diet to make sure you are growing and gaining weight. They teach you about what you should eat and how much. They are also in charge of your pancreatic enzymes.

7. Your **respiratory therapist** teaches you about your airway clearance techniques (see page 19-21). They also teach you about inhaled medications that we use in CF. They will show you what they are used for, how to take them, and in what order to take them.

8. Your **pharmacist** is an expert in medicines and makes sure you are taking all the right ones.

9. Your **psychologist** can help you manage your emotions and/or problems with balancing your treatments. You can talk to them if you feel stressed, angry, or sad.

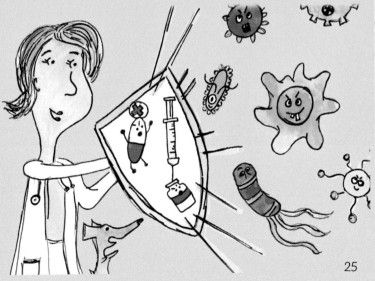

# Doctor Words

**Gene –** a piece of DNA that is passed down to you from your parents; genes carry information that determine all kinds of things about you – like your hair color, your height, and if you have genetic conditions, like CF.

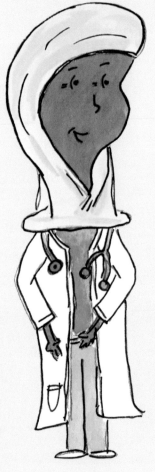

**Gene mutation –** CF is most commonly caused by a mistake, or a gene mutation, in a gene called the CFTR gene (Cystic Fibrosis Transmembrane Conductance Regulator gene).

**Newborn screening –** a special test used to see if newborn babies have CF. It checks your blood to see if you have one of the gene mutations that causes CF.

**Sweat test –** another special test that also checks, in a different way, if a baby has CF. It counts the amount of salt in your sweat. Babies with CF have very salty sweat.

**Exocrine glands –** parts of your body that make sweat, mucus, tears, and pancreatic enzymes. CF can cause problems in all exocrine glands.

**Enzymes –**proteins that help your body function the way it's supposed to; like the pancreatic enzymes that help break down your food!

**Malabsorption –** when your body cannot break down the food you eat. Symptoms of malabsorption include:

a. Poor weight gain

b. Frequent, large, greasy, bad-smelling poops

c. Stomach pain

d. Lots of farting

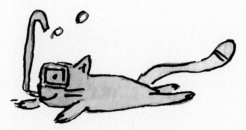

**Mucus plug –** when your thick mucus blocks an opening (like in your lungs, or pancreas).

**Sinusitis –** when your sinus glands get infected and blocked by your thick mucus. This is common in CF and can cause a runny nose and pain or pressure in your face.

**Bronchitis –** when the bronchi of your lungs get blocked by mucus and infected. This is common in CF and can cause fevers and coughs.

**Pneumonia –** this is infection of your lungs that can happen when they get blocked up by mucus. Pneumonia is common in CF and can cause fevers, trouble breathing, and coughing.

**Distal Intestinal Obstructive Syndrome (DIOS) –** when your intestines get blocked by your poop because of the abnormal mucus in your poop. Symptoms include:

a. No (or less) pooping for more than 24 hours

b. Stomach pains

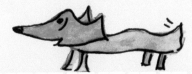

# Meet the Author:
## Dr. Maria Baimas-George

Maria Baimas-George MD MPH is a surgeon, training to specialize in abdominal transplantation. Inspired by her patients and mentors, she writes and illustrates books explaining medical and surgical conditions to children and their loved ones. Her goal is to create books that provide useful information to help with understanding and to offer comfort and hope.

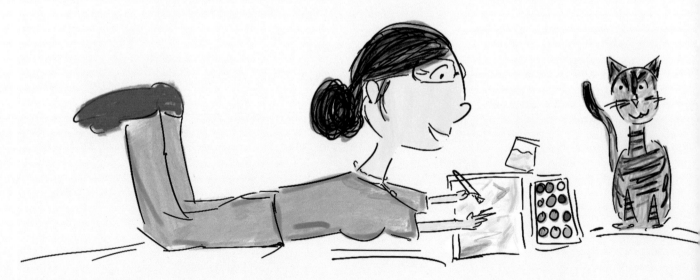